I0782656

Table of Content

Everything You Need to Know About Achalasia

- Causes

- Symptoms

- Diagnosis

- Treatments

- Risk factors

- Outlook

What is Achalasia?

With achalasia, your lower esophageal sphincter (LES) fails to open up during swallowing. This muscular ring closes off your esophagus from your stomach most of the time, but it opens when you swallow so food can pass through. When it doesn't open, food can back up within your esophagus.

Symptoms of this condition tend to come on gradually, and they can get worse as time goes on. Eventually, it can become difficult to swallow liquids or food, but treatment can help.

Who gets achalasia?

In the United States, about 1 in every 100,000 people develop the condition each year

- elsewhere in the world, between 0.1 to 1 in every 100,000 people develop the condition each year

This condition appears to affect people of all genders at roughly the same rates. It's less common in children: Fewer than 5 percentTrusted Source of achalasia cases are diagnosed in children under the age of 16.

While adults of any age can get achalasia, it most commonly develops after age 30 and before age 60.

Is achalasia serious?

Without treatment, achalasia can cause serious health complications, including:

- Megaesophagus. This refers to an enlarged and weakened esophagus.

- Esophagitis. This refers to irritation and inflammation in your esophagus.

- Esophageal perforation. A hole can form in the walls of your esophagus if they become too weak from backed-up food. If this happens, you'll need medical treatment right away to prevent infection.

- Aspiration pneumonia. This happens when the particles of food and liquid trapped in your esophagus enter your lungs

Achalasia can also increase your chances of developing esophageal cancer.

There's no cure for achalasia, so even with treatment, your symptoms may not go away entirely. You may need to have multiple procedures and make permanent lifestyle changes, including:

- eating smaller meals

- avoiding any foods that cause heartburn

- quitting smoking, if you smoke

- sleeping propped up instead of lying flat

Causes

Experts don't know exactly what causes achalasia, though many believe it's caused by a combination of factors, including:

- genetics, or family history

- an autoimmune condition, where your body's immune system mistakenly attacks healthy cells in your body. The degeneration of nerves in your esophagus often contributes to the advanced symptoms of achalasia.

• damage to the nerves in your esophagus or LES

Some have theorizedTrusted Source that viral infections might prompt an autoimmune responses, especially if you have a higher genetic risk of the condition.

Chagas disease, a rare parasitic infection that mostly affects people in Mexico, South America, and Central America, has also been linked to the development of achalasia.

Symptoms

People with achalasia typically experience dysphagia, or trouble swallowing and feeling as if food is stuck in their esophagus. Dysphagia can cause coughing and raise your risk of inhaling and choking on food.

Other possible symptoms include:

• pain or discomfort in your chest

• unexplained weight loss

• heartburn

• intense pain or discomfort after eating

• dry mouth

• dry eyes

You might also have regurgitation or backflow. These symptoms can happen with other gastrointestinal conditions, such as acid reflux. In fact, people with achalasia sometimes first get an incorrect diagnosis of gastroesophageal reflux disease (GERD).

Diagnosis

Achalasia's rarity can complicate diagnosis of the condition, since some doctors may not immediately recognize the signs.

A doctor or other healthcare professional (HCP) might suspect you have achalasia if you:

• have trouble swallowing both solids and liquids and this difficulty worsens over time

• experience regurgitation of food

• have heartburn, chest pain, or both

They may use a few different approaches to help diagnose the condition:

• Endoscopy. In this procedure, a gastroenterologist will insert a tube with a small camera on the end into your esophagus to look for signs of achalasia. This test only leads to diagnosis in about a thirdTrusted Source of achalasia cases, but an endoscopy can help rule out other conditions, like stomach or esophageal cancer.

• X-ray. An X-ray of your chest can show whether your esophagus is enlarged and keeping food trapped inside. A doctor or other HCP may also recommend a barium swallow for the x-ray. Taking liquid barium before your

X-ray makes it possible for them to track how the liquid moves down your esophagus.

- Esophageal manometry (motility study). For this test, a gastroenterologist will pass a narrow tube into your esophagus through your nose. The tube will measure pressure as you swallow, revealing how the muscles of your esophagus work and whether any pressure has built up at the LES.

The order of these diagnostic tests may depend on your specific symptoms and family history, but doctors often recommend an endoscopy first.

Some evidenceTrusted Source suggests esophageal manometry is the most reliable diagnostic tool, as this test can diagnose achalasia more than 90 percent of the time.

Treatment

Achalasia treatment can't completely cure the condition, but it can help:

• improve your ability to swallow by opening the LES

• reduce other symptoms, like pain and regurgitation

• lower the chances of an abnormally enlarged esophagus

Possible treatments include:

Pneumatic dilation

This nonsurgical treatment involves passing a special balloon into the lower part of your esophagus and then inflating it. The balloon helps stretch out the muscles of your LES, expanding the opening so food can pass through more easily.

This procedure isn't without risk, though. Dilation can sometimes lead to esophageal perforation, a fairly uncommon but serious complication. A perforation can be repaired, but if this happens, you'll need surgery right away.

For about 30 percentTrusted Source of people, symptoms will eventually return, so you might need this treatment again in the future.

You're more likely to need repeat treatments if you:

• were assigned male at birth

• are younger than 40 years old

• have respiratory concerns

• have already had the procedure at least once

Botox injections

Another nonsurgical option, this procedure involves injections of botulinum toxin (Botox) into your esophagus during an endoscopy. A doctor or other HCP may recommend this treatment if other treatments don't help or you prefer to avoid surgery.

Botox blocks the nerves that typically signal your muscles to contract, so it can help relax the LES so it opens and allows food to pass through. These injections can improve symptoms quickly. The effects aren't permanent, though, so you'll need to have the treatment repeated within about 6 months to a year.

Potential downsides include the cost of repeated treatments, plus the fact that repeated Botox injections could affect the later success of surgeryTrusted Source.

Laparoscopic Heller myotomy

In a myotomy, a surgeon will cut the LES muscle fibers to help relax it so food can pass into your stomach more easily.

Surgeons can use laparoscopic or robotic techniques to perform this surgery less invasively, through five small incisions to your abdomen. You'll typically need anesthesia and an overnight stay in the hospital.

This surgery has a high success rate, but symptoms of GERD can develop as a possible complication. The surgeon will likely also perform a procedure to help prevent reflux, such as a partial fundoplication.

Peroral endoscopic myotomy

This newer procedure is very similar to a Heller myotomy, but the use of an endoscope makes it less invasive.

The endoscopic approach does have a drawback, though: It prevents the surgeon from doing a partial fundoplication at the same time.

In other words, you have a high risk of experiencing GERD symptoms after the procedure and may need another treatment for GERD later on.

Medication

If you can't get surgery right away, or prefer to avoid it if at all possible, certain medications can offer some relief from your symptoms.

Medication options include:

• nitrates, which help promote relaxation of the smooth muscle making up the lower part of your esophagus

• calcium channel blockers, which can help lower LES pressure by keeping calcium from entering cells and disrupting muscle contractions

- sildenafil, a phosphodiesterase-5 inhibitor that can help lower pressure in the LES, relaxing it enough so food can pass through

These medications may involve some side effects, including:

- low blood pressure

- head pain

- dizziness and fainting

- swelling in your legs and feet

Medications generally won't completely improve your symptoms, either, so a doctor or other HCP will typically only recommend them as a short-term treatment.

Risk factors

Because of achalasia's rarity, experts don't fully understand how or why it occurs, or who might have a greater risk of developing the condition.

A few potential risk factors include:

• having a spinal cord injury

• getting endoscopic sclerotherapy to treat bleeding or enlarged veins

• having a viral infection

• having an autoimmune disease

• age — it's more common in middle age and older adulthood

Future research on achalasia may help experts learn more about possible factors contributing to its development, along with strategies that might help prevent the condition.

Outlook

The outlook for this condition varies. Getting a diagnosis sooner rather than later can help you get treatment to improve your symptoms before they become severe.

You may need multiple treatments before your symptoms improve. Keep in mind, though, that if one treatment doesn't work, you do have other options to consider. A doctor or other HCP might, for example, recommend surgery if a dilation procedure doesn't work.

Older research suggests that while achalasia can cause health complications, it doesn't appear to have a significant impact on life expectancy.

Recipes

How to make the best burgers

Often I see recipes for a burger where all kinds of things are added, include a beaten egg, which I find is really unnecessary.

The best burgers ever are the ones that use the simplest of ingredients and that is good quality ground beef (mince), I don't recommend using any less than 5%

fat ground beef, as otherwise it will just be too lean and dry.

My second tip is to not mix salt into the meat, this tends to draw out the juices of the meat as it cooks and again results in a dry burger.

The best tasting burger is simply just by forming the meat as it is into patties, and season the outside with salt and black pepper just before you add it to a heated pan sprayed with spray oil. Make sure you pan is hot when you add the burgers so that it seals in all the flavour. Then once golden brown flip and cook the other side and the burgers are done.

Can I use other ground meat (mince)?

If you are not a fan of beef, then you can of course use ground chicken or turkey, but the flavour will be slightly different. For me a cheeseburger has to be beef, but that's a personal preference.

Is there a way to make this vegetarian?

If you are vegetarian and want to make this salad, then use one of your favourite vegetarian burgers, brown in a pan and then you can chop up and add to the salad. It will still be delicious.

The perfect low calorie burger salad dressing

No cheeseburger recipe of any kind, be it an actual burger, pasta or quiche etc is complete without a delicious sauce and burger sauce is just the best.

It's so easy to make too and you can reduce the calories by using a mix of light mayonnaise and yoghurt. No one wants a measly drizzle of dressing on th

In my burger sauce I use the follow:

- 3 tablespoons of light mayonnaise

- 1 tablespoon of fat free Greek Yoghurt

- 1 teaspoon of tomato paste (puree)

- 1 teaspoon of American yellow mustard

- ½ teaspoon of sweet paprika

- ¼ teaspoon of garlic powder

- ¼ teaspoon of onion powder

- Pinch of black pepper

- 1 teaspoon of granulated sweetener (optional)

- little water to loosen

Prep Ahead

This is great for preparing in advance too for lunches on the go, packed lunches etc.

Just put the burgers and salad in a container and then store the croutons and dressing in separate containers, then you can add with the croutons and drizzle with the sauce/dressing just before eating.

If you prefer to have the burgers heated and have access to a microwave, you can just warm them up in a the microwave.

Crustless Mushroom Quiche

yield: SERVES 6

prep time: 10 MINUTES

cook time: 1 HOUR

total time: 1 HOUR 10 MINUTES

Crustless Mushroom Quiche - a simple but delicious crustless quiche that is perfect for quick and easy lunches.

4.8 Stars (4 Reviews)

PRINT

Ingredients

- Low calorie cooking spray

- 500g of mushrooms (I used cremini), chopped

- 1 onion, quartered and sliced thinly

- 4 cloves of garlic, crushed

- salt and pepper to season

- 90g of parmesan, freshly grated

- 2 spring onions, finely sliced

- 7 large eggs

- 225g of fat free Greek Yoghurt

-

Instructions

1. Preheat oven to 180c, fan 160c, 350f or gas mark 4

2. Spray a frying pan over a medium high heat with low calorie cooking spray.

3. Fry onions and mushrooms until lightly browned (approx 9 minutes)

4. Add the garlic and a pinch of salt and black pepper and fry for a further minute.

5. Whisk eggs with the yoghurt until well combined.

6. Grease a 8 inch springform pan lined with parchment paper with low calorie cooking spray, then pour in the egg and yoghurt mixture.

7. Add the mushroom mixture, along with the spring onion and parmesan, roughly combine with a spatula, leaving some of the parmesan on top.

8. Bake in the oven for approx 45 minutes until lightly golden and set.

9. Allow to cool slightly before remove from springform pan and slicing.

10. Enjoy!!

Crustless Mushroom Quiche

yield: SERVES 6

prep time: 10 MINUTES

cook time: 1 HOUR

total time: 1 HOUR 10 MINUTES

Crustless Mushroom Quiche - a simple but delicious crustless quiche that is perfect for quick and easy lunches.

4.8 Stars (4 Reviews)

PRINT

Ingredients

- Low calorie cooking spray

- 500g of mushrooms (I used cremini), chopped

- 1 onion, quartered and sliced thinly

- 4 cloves of garlic, crushed

- salt and pepper to season

- 90g of parmesan, freshly grated

- 2 spring onions, finely sliced

- 7 large eggs

- 225g of fat free Greek Yoghurt

-

Instructions

1. Preheat oven to 180c, fan 160c, 350f or gas mark 4

2. Spray a frying pan over a medium high heat with low calorie cooking spray.

3. Fry onions and mushrooms until lightly browned (approx 9 minutes)

4. Add the garlic and a pinch of salt and black pepper and fry for a further minute.

5. Whisk eggs with the yoghurt until well combined.

6. Grease a 8 inch springform pan lined with parchment paper with low calorie cooking spray, then pour in the egg and yoghurt mixture.

7. Add the mushroom mixture, along with the spring onion and parmesan, roughly combine with a spatula, leaving some of the parmesan on top.

8. Bake in the oven for approx 45 minutes until lightly golden and set.

9. Allow to cool slightly before remove from springform

pan and slicing.

10. Enjoy!!

Southwestern Turkey Meatballs | Slimming Friendly

yield: SERVES 4

prep time: 15 MINUTES

cook time: 45 MINUTES

total time: 1 HOUR

Southwestern Turkey Meatballs - delicious turkey meatballs in a amazing spicy Southwestern Style Sauce with black beans, corn and veggies

PRINT

Ingredients

For the meatballs:

- 500g (17.5oz) of Extra Lean Ground Turkey or Chicken

- ⅓ cup of breadcrumbs (30g)

- pinch of onion powder

- pinch of garlic powder

- 1 tablespoons of tomato paste

- salt and black pepper

- 1 egg, beaten

For the sauce:

- 1 onion, finely chopped

- 1 carrot, finely chopped

- 2 cloves of garlic, crushed

- 1 jalapeno, chopped (seeds removed)

- 1 red pepper, finely chopped

- 1 green pepper finely chopped

- 2 teaspoons of cumin

- 2 teaspoons of paprika

- 1 teaspoon of oregano

- pinch of cayenne pepper - add more or less depending on how spicy you like it.

- 2 teaspoons of sweetener - I use erythritol

- 1 cup (240g) of passata

- 3 tablespoons of tomato paste

- 2 cups (480ml) of chicken stock

- 160g of sweetcorn (canned), drained

- 200g black beans (canned), drained and rinsed

- fresh coriander

- cooking oil spray

- salt and black pepper

Instructions

1. Preheat oven to 200c, 180c fan, 400f or gas mark 6

2. In a bowl add the ground turkey, breadcrumbs, onion powder, garlic powder, tomato paste, salt, black pepper and egg.

3. Work together well, then form into 16 meatballs

4. Place meatballs on a baking tray lined with parchment paper, spray over the top with spray oil and bake for 10-15 minutes until lightly golden and set aside.

5. Spray a deep large frying pan over a medium high heat with cooking oil spray, add the onion, and carrot and fry for approx 5 mins until softened.

6. Add the garlic, peppers, and jalapeno and fry for a few more minutes.

7. Add the spices, passata, tomato paste, sweetener and stock, bring to a boil.

8. Reduce heat, add back in the meatballs along with the black beans and sweet corn and simmer for 20-30 minutes until the sauce reduces down and thickens.

9. Sprinkle with chopped coriander and season with salt and black pepper as needed.

10. Serve and enjoy!!

Roasted Garlic Hummus

yield: SERVES 4

prep time: 10 MINUTES

cook time: 55 MINUTES

total time: 1 HOUR 5 MINUTES

Delicious creamy hummus with the amazing flavours of roasted garlic for a perfect dip to enjoy for lunch or as a snack

4.5 Stars (11 Reviews)

PRINT

Ingredients

For the Hummus:

- 1 400g can of chickpeas, including liquid

- 1 small bulb of garlic (whole bulb)

- 1 teaspoon of ground cumin

- 1 teaspoon of paprika (not smoked)

- juice of a whole lemon

- 1 tablespoon of tahini paste

- water

- sea salt to taste

For the topping:

- pinch of paprika

- pinch of fine sea salt

- fresh chopped parsley

- 1 teaspoons of olive oil

Instructions

1. Preheat oven to 200c (180c fan), 400f or gas mark 6

1. Slice the top of the bulb of garlic, so it just exposes the tips of all the cloves, spray the exposed garlic with olive oil spray,

2. Wrap up in foil, place in a baking dish and roast for approx 40-50 minutes. You want the garlic to be really soft and caramelized (but don't burn). Allow to cool slightly

3. Squeeze the roasted garlic out of the bulb and add to a food processor with the chickpeas (including liquid), juice of a lemon, cumin, paprika, garlic, tahini paste and blend or food process until a smooth consistency, if needed add in a little bit of water at a time to help blending process.

4. Once smooth, taste and season with salt to required taste.

5. Add to a bowl, smooth over the top, creating a few peaks as you do. Sprinkle with a pinch of paprika, some coarse sea salt and then drizzle with the 1 teaspoon of extra virgin olive oil. Finish off with a little fresh chopped parsley.

6. Dig in and enjoy!!

7. Store Hummus in a airtight container in the fridge, it should keep for about 5-7 days.

Beef and Pinto Bean Chilli

yield: SERVES 6

prep time: 15 MINUTES

cook time: 1 HOUR

total time: 1 HOUR 15 MINUTES

There is nothing quite as comforting as a delicious bowl of chilli with all the toppings and this yummy beef and pinto bean chilli is both rich in flavours and hearty and filling. It will become a regular meal for the whole family

5.0 Stars (2 Reviews)

PRINT

Ingredients

- 1 large onion, finely diced

- 2 stalks of celery, diced

- 1 large carrot, diced

- 455g (1lb) of 5% fat ground beef (beef mince)

- 3 cloves of garlic, minced

- 1 tablespoon of paprika

- 1 tablespoon of cumin

- ½ tablespoon of oregano

- ½ tablespoon of chipotle chilli powder (do not use Indian chilli powder)

- ½ tablespoon of brown sugar

- 1 teaspoon of onion powder

- ½ teaspoon of cayenne pepper

- 8 tablespoons of tomato puree (paste)

- 1 red pepper, finely diced

- 1 yellow or orange pepper, finely diced

- 2 jalapenos, deseeded and diced

- 2 x 400g (14oz) cans of chopped tomatoes

- 1 cup (240ml) of chicken stock

- 1 x 400g (14oz) can of pinto beans, drained

- cooking oil spray

- salt and black pepper

- 2 spring onions (green onions), diced

Instructions

1. Spray a large saucepan over a medium heat with spray oil

2. Add the onion, celery, carrot and a pinch of sea salt and fry until softened (approx 5 minutes) - add in a little water to prevent burning if needed.

1. Add the beef mince, garlic and red and orange bell pepper and continue to fry until the beef is browned.

2. Add the tomato puree (paste), sugar and all the spices and mix until well coated.

3. Add the canned chopped tomatoes, pinto beans, jalapeño and stock, bring to the boil and cover and simmer for approx 45 minutes until sauce reduces and thickens. (If liquid reduces too much you can add in a little more stock or water)

4. Once cooked, taste and season well with salt and

pepper to taste and sprinkle with the chopped spring

onion.

Chicken Meatballs in Hoisin Sauce

yield: SERVES 4

prep time: 10 MINUTES

cook time: 30 MINUTES

total time: 40 MINUTES

Chicken Meatballs in Hoisin Sauce - delicious juicy chicken meatballs with mushrooms in a rich flavour packed Hoisin Sauce.

4.6 Stars (58 Reviews)

PRINT

Ingredients

For the meatballs:

- 500g extra lean ground chicken (mince) - 5% fat

- 125g of mushrooms

- 1 garlic clove, minced

- ½ tsp of ginger root

- pinch of salt and pepper

For the sauce:

- 3 tablespoons of hoisin sauce

- 3 tablespoons of dark soy sauce (use low sodium soy sauce if you prefer)

- 2 tablespoon of tomato paste (puree)

- 180ml (¾ cup) of water

- 180ml (¾ cup) of passata

- 1 tablespoon of cornstarch (cornflour)

- ½ teaspoon of garlic powder

- ½ teaspoon of onion powder

To Serve:

- 3 spring onions (green onions), sliced

- pinch of black and toasted sesame seeds

Instructions

1. Preheat oven to 200c, 180c fan or 400f (gas mark 6)

2. Add the mushrooms, garlic and ginger to a mini food processor and pulse until really fine.

3. Add this to a bowl with the chicken mince and a pinch of salt and black pepper and combine all together.

4. Form into 16 equal sized meatballs

5. Place meatballs on a baking tray lined with parchment, spray over top with cooking oil spray and bake for approx 10-15 minutes until lightly golden.

6. Whisk together the sauce ingredients

7. Add to a frying pan and drop in the meatballs.

8. Let sauce bubble until sauce reduces down and thickens and meatballs are cooked through. (approx 10-15 minutes)

9. Serve topped with sliced spring onion and a pinch of black and toasted sesame seeds.

10. Enjoy!!

Asparagus Soup

yield: SERVES 4

prep time: 10 MINUTES

cook time: 20 MINUTES

total time: 30 MINUTES

Dig in and enjoy a bowl of this delicious Asparagus Soup which feels indulgent and creamy but is made from the simplest of ingredients.

4.5 Stars (36 Reviews)

PRINT

Ingredients

- 1 large onion, finely chopped

- 1 leek, sliced

- 1 clove of garlic, minced

- 600g of asparagus spears (chopped), tough ends broken off

- some fresh thyme leaves

- 4 cups (960ml) of chicken or vegetable stock

- salt and pepper to season

- olive oil spray

Instructions

1. Spray a large saucepan over a medium heat with some cooking oil spray

2. Add the onion, leek and garlic cook until softened.

3. Add some fresh thyme and asparagus

4. Add the stock and bring to a boil. Reduce heat cover and simmer until Asparagus is tender (approx 15 mins).

5. Remove half the mixture and blend (or blend the whole soup if you prefer), then return to the pan, stir

and just simmer for a further few mins until it's lovely

and silky in appear

6. Taste and season with salt and black pepper

7. Enjoy

Notes

Please see below for recipe values:

This recipe is gluten free, dairy free, vegetarian, paleo,

Whole30 friendly

• Slimming World - syn free per serving

• WW Personal Points - 0 per serving (add ingredients

to your WW diary for points value - as this may vary

depending on your personal points zero foods)

- Vegetarian - use vegetable stock

- Gluten Free - use gluten free stock

Sweet Potato, Vegetable and Lentil Chilli

yield: SERVES 8

prep time: 10 MINUTES

cook time: 2 HOURS

total time: 2 HOURS 10 MINUTES

Enjoy a comforting and filling bowl of Sweet Potato, Vegetable and Lentil Chilli with some of your favourite toppings.

4.5 Stars (76 Reviews)

PRINT

Ingredients

- 1 onion, finely chopped

- 1 red pepper, finely chopped

- 2 jalapeno's, deseeded and chopped

- 1 courgette finely chopped

- 1 small carrot, finely chopped

- 2 cloves of garlic crushed

- 1 stalk of celery, chopped

- 300g (10.5oz) of cubed sweet potato

- 190g (1 cup) of uncooked green lentils (can also used brown)

- 4 ripe medium tomatoes, peeled and chopped (can use canned, but drain of excess liquid)

- 720ml (3 cups) of chicken or vegetable stock

- 240g (1 cup) of passata

- 2 tablespoon of tomato paste (puree)

- 1 tablespoon of Mexican chilli/chili powder - see note*

- 2 teaspoons of cumin

- 2 teaspoons of paprika

- 1 teaspoon of oregano

- pinch of cayenne (optional if you like it hot)

- splash of balsamic vinegar

- spray oil

Instructions

1. Spray a large saucepan with spray oil.

2. Add the onion, garlic, celery, carrot and fry till softened.

3. Add the courgette, vine tomatoes, red pepper, jalapeno, sweet potato.

4. Add in spices and stir to coat.

5. Pour in the stock, passata, tomato puree and lentils and bring to the boil.

6. Add a splash of balsamic vinegar, reduce the heat, cover, and simmer for approx 1.5 – 2 hours, lentils

should be nice and tender.. If you prefer the courgette

firmer, add this in for the last 30 minutes of cooking

instead

7. Taste and season as needed with salt and black

pepper.

8. Serve with your choice of sides/toppings

9. Enjoy!!

Spicy Garlic Napa Cabbage

yield: SERVES 4

prep time: 10 MINUTES

cook time: 10 MINUTES

total time: 20 MINUTES

Spicy Garlic Napa Cabbage - delicious pan fried Napa cabbage with fresh garlic and the spicy kick from red chilli flakes. A perfect side for a variety of main dishes.

4.8 Stars (5 Reviews)

PRINT

Ingredients

- 1 medium sized Napa cabbage, roughly chopped

- 3 cloves of garlic, minced

- 4 spring onions (green onions), chopped

- 1 teaspoon of red chilli flakes

- 1.5 tablespoons of soy sauce (I used Kikkoman)

- ¼ cup (60ml) of water

- 2 teaspoons of maple syrup

- 1 teaspoon of toasted sesame oil

- pinch of white pepper

- spray oil

Instructions

1. Heat a frying pan over a medium high heat, spray with cooking oil spray add the garlic and fry for about 30 secs to infuse flavour/soften. (be careful not to burn)

2. Add in the cabbage with the soy sauce, red chilli flakes, pinch of white pepper and a ¼ cup of water.

3. Cook until the cabbage softens and most of the liquid

is cooked off, then add in the green onions, sesame oil

and maple syrup and continue to cook until the liquid

left in the pan coats the cabbage in a slightly glossy

sauce.

4. Serve with your favourite main course.

5. Enjoy!!

Spicy Garlic Napa Cabbage

yield: SERVES 4

prep time: 10 MINUTES

cook time: 10 MINUTES

total time: 20 MINUTES

Spicy Garlic Napa Cabbage - delicious pan fried Napa cabbage with fresh garlic and the spicy kick from red chilli flakes. A perfect side for a variety of main dishes.

4.8 Stars (5 Reviews)

PRINT

Ingredients

- 1 medium sized Napa cabbage, roughly chopped

- 3 cloves of garlic, minced

- 4 spring onions (green onions), chopped

- 1 teaspoon of red chilli flakes

- 1.5 tablespoons of soy sauce (I used Kikkoman)

- ¼ cup (60ml) of water

- 2 teaspoons of maple syrup

- 1 teaspoon of toasted sesame oil

- pinch of white pepper

- spray oil

Instructions

1. Heat a frying pan over a medium high heat, spray with cooking oil spray add the garlic and fry for about 30 secs to infuse flavour/soften. (be careful not to burn)

2. Add in the cabbage with the soy sauce, red chilli flakes, pinch of white pepper and a ¼ cup of water.

3. Cook until the cabbage softens and most of the liquid is cooked off, then add in the green onions, sesame oil and maple syrup and continue to cook until the liquid left in the pan coats the cabbage in a slightly glossy sauce.

4. Serve with your favourite main course.

5. Enjoy!!

Korean Ground Pork

yield: SERVES 4

prep time: 10 MINUTES

cook time: 20 MINUTES

total time: 30 MINUTES

Korean Ground Pork - super easy to make and packed with flavour. Perfect with a simple side or make it a bowl with a variety of yummy components.

4.5 Stars (47 Reviews)

PRINT

Ingredients

- 455g (1lb) of extra lean ground pork (can also use chicken, turkey or beef)

- 1 onion, finely diced

- 3 cloves of garlic, minced

- 1 tablespoon of grated ginger root

- 2 tablespoon of Gochujang Paste (use 1 if you don't like food too spicy)

- 2 tablespoon of soy sauce

- 2 tablespoons of maple syrup or honey

- ¼ cup of water

- 1 teaspoon of toasted sesame oil

- pinch of sesame seeds

- 2 green onions (spring onions) sliced

- Spray oil

Instructions

1. Add the ground pork to a frying pan over a medium

high heat and cook until browned, breaking up any

large clumps as it cooks. Remove and set aside.

2. Spray the pan with cooking oil spray, add the onion

and fry until lightly golden and softened.

3. Add in the garlic and ginger and fry for a further

minute.

4. Add back in the ground pork, along with the

Gochujang paste, soy sauce, maple syrup and sesame

oil and water and cook until it reduces down and coats

all the ground pork and starts to caramelize on the

edges.

5. Sprinkle with a pinch of toasted sesame seeds and chopped green onions

6. Serve with your favourite sides.

7. Enjoy!!!

Fruity Chicken Curry

yield: SERVES 4

prep time: 10 MINUTES

cook time: 40 MINUTES

total time: 50 MINUTES

Fruity Chicken Curry - a delicious curry with tender pieces of chicken in a flavoursome curry sauce with vegetables and the sweetness from sultanas and the juice of an orange make it the perfect family recipe.

4.5 Stars (69 Reviews)

PRINT

Ingredients

• 6 uncooked boneless skinless chicken thighs, trimmed of visible fat and sliced into bite size pieces (approx 600g/21oz)

• 1 medium courgette (zucchini), chopped

• 1 medium carrot, chopped

- 1 onion, finely chopped

- 2 cloves of garlic, crushed

- 1 teaspoon of fresh grated ginger

- juice of an orange

- 30g (1oz) of sultanas

- 2 teaspoons of ground cumin

- 2 teaspoons of ground coriander

- 1 teaspoon of medium chilli powder

- 1 teaspoon of mustard seeds

- ½ teaspoon of turmeric

- ½ teaspoon of garam masala

- 1 cup (240ml) of chicken stock/broth

- 2 tablespoons of tomato paste (puree)

- Spray oil

- Salt and black pepper

- fresh coriander to serve

Instructions

1. Spray a frying pan over a medium high heat with some spray oil.

2. Add the mustard seeds and once they start to pop, add the onion, carrot, ginger and garlic.

3. Cook for a couple of mins until they start to go golden.

4. Add the turmeric, cumin, coriander and chilli powder and stir to coat

5. Add the chicken and a pinch of salt and black pepper and fry until browned.

6. Add the courgette (zucchini), stock, tomato paste, juice of half an orange, sultanas and garam masala and bring to the boil, reduce heat slightly and simmer for approx 25-30 minutes until sauce has reduced and chicken is lovely and tender.

7. Taste and season with salt and black pepper as needed.

8. Serve topped with some fresh coriander and your choice of sides.

9. Enjoy!!

Homemade Pickled Red Onions

yield: SERVES 8

prep time: 15 MINUTES

cook time: 5 MINUTES

total time: 20 MINUTES

Pickled Red Onions - an easy simple recipe for homemade pickled red onion, once you try these you will never buy store bought again. Perfect condiment to a variety of dishes.

4.5 Stars (17 Reviews)

PRINT

Ingredients

- 250g (9oz) of red onion, sliced thinly

- 120ml (½ cup) of white vinegar

- 120ml (½ cup) of red wine vinegar

- 240ml (1 cup) of water

- 3 tablespoons of white sugar (or use any sweetener of your choice)

- 2 cloves of garlic, sliced thinly

- ½ teaspoon of dried oregano

- 1 teaspoon of dried dill

- 2 teaspoons of fine sea salt

Instructions

1. Remove peel from onions, and using a sharp knife or mandolin slice thinly. Set aside.

2. Heat the vinegar and water, with the sugar and salt in a small saucepan until the sugar is fully dissolved and then set aside to cool.

3. Add the onions to a large container or jar (you can use two if you don't have a large one big enough).

4. Once the pickling liquid has cooled, add in the sliced garlic, dried dill and oregano and stir until all combined.

5. Pour this oven the onions, ensuring the onions are all pushed down and submerged in the pickling juice.

6. Keep in a. airtight container/jar in fridge. I find these

are best left for the flavour to develop overnight before

enjoying for the first time.